T0054266

101 ways to be
less stressed

101 ways to be
less stressed

Simple Self-Care Strategies to
Boost Your **MIND, MOOD,**
and **MENTAL HEALTH**

DR. CAROLINE LEAF

BakerBooks

a division of Baker Publishing Group
Grand Rapids, Michigan

Published by Baker Books
a division of Baker Publishing Group
PO Box 6287, Grand Rapids, MI 49516-6287
www.bakerbooks.com

Printed in the United States of America

Library of Congress Cataloging-in-Publication Data
Names: Leaf, Caroline, 1963– author.
Title: 101 ways to be less stressed : simple self-care strategies to
    boost your mind, mood, and mental health / Caroline Leaf.
Other titles: One hundred one ways to be less stressed
Description: Grand Rapids, Michigan : Baker Books, a division of
    Baker Publishing Group, 2020.
Identifiers: LCCN 2020015831 | ISBN 9781540900937 (cloth)
Subjects: LCSH: Stress management—Popular works. | Self-care,
    Health—Popular works.
Classification: LCC RA785 .L43 2020 | DDC 155.9/042—dc23
LC record available at https://lccn.loc.gov/2020015831

This publication is intended to provide helpful and informative
material on the subjects addressed.
Readers should consult their personal
health professionals before adopting
any of the suggestions in this book
or drawing inferences from it. The
author and publisher expressly disclaim
responsibility for any adverse effects
arising from the use or application of
the information contained in this book.

In keeping with biblical principles of
creation stewardship, Baker Publishing Group advocates the responsible
use of our natural resources. As a
member of the Green Press Initia-
tive, our company uses recycled
paper when possible. The text paper
of this book is composed in part of
post-consumer waste.

23 24 25 26   7 6 5

introduction

Although many of us spend time focusing on our physical health, whether it's going to the gym, to a Pilates class, or for a morning jog, we often forget to work on our mental health. Yet the mind is the source of all our thoughts, words, and actions; when our thinking is unhealthy, our life will be unhealthy—even if we work out seven times a week and eat kale every day.

It's very important to spend time focusing on our mental self-care regimen and ways to be less stressed, since mental toughness and resilience will get us through difficult times and help us achieve success in every area of life, as I discuss in my book *Think, Learn, Succeed*. When our mind is strong, we'll be able to handle whatever life throws our way; we can go from surviving to thriving.

Of course, life can be very challenging. We're constantly facing stressful situations at work, at home, at school, in the car . . . you name it! In many cases, our reactions to these situations can make things worse. If we let our thoughts and emotions get the best of us, we can negatively impact both our mental and physical well-being. Uncontrolled thoughts and emotions run rampant through our brain, creating neurochemical chaos that can make us anxious, affecting our ability to think clearly and process information. This is one of the major roadblocks to success and can allow other toxic thinking habits and mental health issues to take root.

Here's the good news: our mind is incredibly powerful and incredibly capable. Our brain can change as we think (neuroplasticity) and grow new brain cells (neurogenesis). Using the incredible power in our mind, we can persist and grow in response to life's challenges. We can take our thoughts captive and change the way we think, speak, and act.

Our minds are more than prepared to stand up to these trials and overcome them—all we have to do is *think well*. Mentally healthy people can handle all of life's challenges. By changing our thinking and living a life of mental self-care, we can improve the way we think and how we live.

This book was created as a guide to help you understand the unique power of your mind, your choices, and your impact. It is, essentially, a beginner's how-to guide to mental self-care. It's a guide to 101 simple self-care strategies to boost your mind, mood, and mental health. As you reflect on each tip, I recommend the following process: *ask, answer*, and *discuss*.

These three actions underscore the intentional and deliberate process of learning that produces intelligent memory, which goes beyond merely reading some information you will forget later (for more on learning and memory formation, see my book *Think, Learn, Succeed*).

First, *ask*. In a journal, write down several questions about the tip you've read. For example, you can ask yourself, *Have I ever felt that I wasn't good enough? That I couldn't cope with the circumstances of life? How did I respond? What effect did this have in my life?* Your questions are meant to provide a starting point for an internal dialogue, much like questions you and I would ask each other during a day-to-day conversation.

Next, *answer*. Here you apply the tip to your own life by responding, in detail, to your questions in the *ask* section. It is important to remember that there are no right or wrong answers in this section. You answer your own questions, which are shaped by your experiences and the unique way you think, feel, and choose (see my book *The Perfect You* for more information).

Finally, *discuss*. In your journal, you further examine your own thoughts, words, and actions, considering the mental self-care tip of the day, expanding your observations, and thinking of practical ways you can change your mind and change your life.

So, are you interested in learning how to use the incredible power of your mind to persist and grow in response to life's challenges? No matter what life throws your way, when you master the art of mental self-care, you will boost your mind, mood, and mental health and achieve success in life.

1| Set your intentions for the week

At the beginning of each week, set your intentions for the week, including some time for fun and for "thinker moments," when you switch off to the external and switch on to the internal to just let your mind wander and meditate. This will help you mentally prepare for the week ahead, help you build up stress resilience, and give you time to organize your thinking. What are your intentions for this week? When is the right time for you to set your intentions for each week?

2| Be open and honest with your intentions

The majority of arguments and misunderstandings happen because you and I are not clear or honest about how we feel or what we want, either because we expect others to just know what we want or we're afraid to be open about how we feel. The solution: practice being open, clear, and honest about your intentions while being gentle and kind. What are some of your intentions that you could communicate to those you love?

3| Learn what your body needs and make it a priority

The gut microbiome—the world of bacteria living in the digestive system—doesn't just exist to help us break down food. There's a constant conversation going on between the brain and the gut, which has its own amazing neurons, just like the spinal cord. The relationship between the gut and the brain is incredibly important when it comes to mental health. So make your gut health a priority by listening to your body and watching what you eat.

4| When you are panicking about something, focus your attention on one thing

When you're panicking, find a single object to focus all your attention on. Pick one thing in clear sight and consciously and deliberately note everything about it you possibly can: describe the patterns, color, shape, and size of the object to yourself. Focus all your energy on this object to help control the symptoms of panic.

5| Incorporate more "thinker moments" into your day

When you take time to switch off to the external and switch on to the internal and just let your mind wander, you boost your brain health. These "thinker moments" give your brain a rest and allow it to reboot and heal by letting your mind wander and daydream, which increases clarity of mind and the ability to problem-solve. So be intentional about creating daily "thinker" breaks throughout your day, or when you're feeling stressed out, to switch off and just focus on the internal by taking a few minutes to sit and daydream or meditate. How will you start incorporating more "thinker moments" in your schedule?

6 | Avoid claiming panic attacks as part of your identity

Never say "my panic attacks," as claiming them as your identity can become a self-fulfilling prophecy, since whatever you think about and believe in grows stronger in your brain, affecting what you say and do. Just see them as a reaction, like an allergy. Don't live into the identity of associating yourself with panic attacks.

7| Take a warm bath or shower before bed

If you battle falling asleep, this tip is for you. Recent research has shown a warm shower or bath before bed can improve both sleep quality and ease of falling asleep.

8| Get creative

Feeling depressed, anxious, or just stuck in a rut? Force yourself to do something creative. Creativity boosts confidence; allows for more "thinker moments," which are vital for mental health; and enhances imagination, which helps with problem-solving and troubleshooting everyday life issues! So, try out new hobbies and include more time in your schedule for creativity. Some easy ideas include keeping a coloring book on your desk, doodling, writing, composing, painting, cooking, baking, or building a puzzle.

9| How to keep your brain young and healthy

1. Detox your mind, brain, and body daily.

2. Build your brain daily.

3. Get enough sleep.

10| Make sure you are getting enough omegas

Omegas are vital for brain health because they help build and strengthen our myelin sheath, which enables us to think about and process information at much faster speeds and with more efficiency. This, in turn, increases our cognitive performance, boosting our mental and physical health by positively impacting the way our brain and body function on a day-to-day basis. Try to include more omega-rich foods in your diet, such as wild and sustainable salmon, flaxseeds, chia seeds, walnuts, and so on.

11| Be aware of your thoughts

When you're aware of a problem in your life, you can strengthen or weaken that issue based on the choices you make. You can choose to ruminate on the problem, allowing a toxic thought structure to grow in your brain and impact your mental and physical health and relationships. Or you can choose to deal with the issue by acknowledging and embracing it, talking through it with someone, finding triggers, and having an action plan in place to resolve the issue. Don't ruminate on a problem; reconceptualize the issue. This means looking at it as an opportunity to grow, learn, develop, and build up your stress resilience.

12| Practice deep breathing

As soon as you start feeling depressed, anxious, worried, fearful, or panicked, practice deep breathing, which helps reduce cortisol levels in the brain and body that are blocking your cognition, allowing you to decompress. Hyperventilating can make you feel worse, while deep, slow breathing calms you down, reducing levels of adrenaline and cortisol and allowing your HPA axis (which controls the stress reaction) to work for you and not against you, preparing you for positive action. One technique to control your breathing

I highly recommend (and use often!) is to breathe in deeply for four seconds, hold for four seconds, and breathe out for four seconds. You can also breathe in one side of your nose and out the other side, which also helps you decompress.

13| Engage in conversation with people who have different points of view

One great way to actively build your brain is to engage in conversation with people who have different opinions and beliefs. You'll not only learn more but your brain will have to work extra hard to process the information. This mental stimulation is great for both your physical and mental health. Just remember to always listen without judgment, pride, arrogance, or condemnation. Listen and speak with the aim to learn and grow.

14| Practice "purposeful procrastination"

Practicing "purposeful procrastination" may be one way to reduce unnecessary anxiety in your life. It means learning to accept incompleteness: you can't always get everything done at once, so you should clear a space in your mind and compartmentalize, setting aside other tasks for later. Be okay with saying no and not getting something done immediately. You may also need to reevaluate the deadlines you place on yourself, as these may be unrealistic and cause you more stress than necessary. Are there places in your life where you feel you can do this?

15| Red light therapy can potentially help improve your mental and physical health

Numerous studies have shown that red light therapy is *one* way we can help heal and improve our mental, cognitive, and physical health. Of course, as I have said many times before, there is no "magic bullet" when it comes to our mind and brain. Living a life of mental self-care means paying attention to all aspects of our mental and physical health, including what we think, what we eat, our sleeping patterns, how much we exercise, and so on. And, as part of this balanced, mind-centered approach to living well, red light therapy can be a real plus. The spectrum of light associated with red light therapy has the unique ability to stimulate our cells, in particular our mitochondria (the powerhouses of our cells), which creates more energy in the body through increased adenosine triphosphate production, allowing it to function on a higher level. This enhanced mitochondrial function and increased blood flow can potentially lead to reduced inflammation, better sleeping patterns, healthier-looking skin, improved muscle recovery, less joint pain, better moods, enhanced memory, and much more.

16| Be careful of relying too much on "self-help"

In many cases, the self-help industry is problematic because it promotes the idea that to be better we should focus only on ourselves. This goes against our biology and the design of our brain: we need each other to be better, and we need each other to heal. While it's of course important to work on ourselves and our mental, physical, and emotional health, we should also be intentional about our "social health." Think of ways you can be intentional about building community: start a volunteer group or a book club, go to talk therapy, or help someone you know who is hurting. The opportunities are endless.

17| Walk more

Looking for a quick stress release, an
antidote to anxiety, or a creativity boost?
Go for a walk outside. Fresh air, nature,
and physical movement are some of the
best antidepressants.

18| Give yourself time to forgive

If you've been hurt by someone, don't be too hard on yourself if you can't immediately forgive them and move on. Don't try to "fake it till you make it" when it comes to forgiveness, because you can't just get rid of, pray away, or suppress feelings or emotions, which are physical structures in the brain that will take time and effort to break down. Healing takes time. Be compassionate and patient with yourself. Start by acknowledging your feelings, recognizing you want them to go away, and then using mental self-care techniques like reconceptualization (reimagining your thoughts) to detox your brain. It also helps to talk to someone about your feelings and/or write them down—this will help you gain clarity and perspective.

19| Sometimes it's better to focus on facts rather than emotions

Learning to embrace negative thoughts or emotions can be incredibly uncomfortable, but it's necessary in order to overcome whatever is causing them. To make this process a little easier, don't just focus on how you feel; rather, focus on the facts or logic of the situation and ask yourself questions. For example, maybe you got an email that caused you to feel stressed and anxious. Instead of thinking about how you feel and panicking, focus on the words of the email. What is this person saying? Why did it make you feel stressed and anxious? What are the facts of the situation? Could this person be right, and you are overreacting? Is there something in this situation that you can learn from? Are you basing your thinking on assumptions or on facts? If you keep practicing this consistently, focusing on facts will become a habit and help reduce anxiety in your life.

20| Don't suppress your anxiety

Anxiety is often a symptom of unexplored and suppressed emotions. When you feel something negative or something you think is stupid or embarrassing, don't suppress or ignore it. Embrace it, learn from it, and reconceptualize it.

21 | Improve your nutrition and boost your mental health

Here are three simple nutrition tips to help boost your brain and mental health:

1. Eat sitting down.

2. Work on improving the health of your gut microbiome, such as by taking probiotics and eating low-sugar foods.

3. Reduce or eliminate processed and refined sugars and carbs.

22| Acceptance is important

Confidence often comes from accepting external factors you can't control. Learning to accept your emotional reactions and feedback, and to "metabolize" them, is key to increasing your confidence. Some ways you can start to do this is by becoming aware of and embracing situations where you can be vulnerable, seeking feedback no matter what, and reconceptualizing all negative feedback or emotions as opportunities to grow and learn. What can you start learning to accept today?

23| Work on your insecurities

If you struggle with jealousy, insecurity, or envy (which the majority of us do), it may be helpful to remember:

1. Life is not a zero-sum game. Just because someone is doing well does not mean there is less of a chance you will do well; there is no "success reservoir" that is being depleted. The more we all succeed, the more we all benefit—the bigger the pie gets, the more people get a slice.

2. Don't get stuck in the shame and guilt associated with these feelings. Rather, acknowledge them (tell yourself it is great you are aware of them) and then see what they are telling you. Maybe you need to improve in a certain area of your life? Maybe you need to address something deeper? It is always important to work through uncomfortable emotions—never suppress them.

24| Don't let your failures define you

Do you confuse failure as an action with failure as an identity? Too often we cause ourselves mental distress because we see failure as a part of us or a part of someone else. Rather, we need to look at failure as an external action outside of an identity, like stumbling: it happened to us, but we just get back up again. When we make failure a part of our identity, we make it more permanent. Be careful of saying that you're a failure or someone else is a failure. It's far better to say, "I failed, but that is in the past" and focus on what you learned from the situation. See failure as a verb, not an adjective—an action, not a description.

25| Be careful of basing your words and actions on assumptions

Constantly check that what you think, say, and do are not just based on assumptions. Do you have all the facts? If not, your assumptions are essentially building structures into your brain and creating realities made of half-truths, misinformation, and, in many cases, lies, which will negatively impact your mental health.

26| Watch how you judge situations

Often a situation itself does not cause mental distress. Rather, it's our judgment of that situation that causes us mental pain or pleasure. We need to constantly be aware of how we're perceiving and judging situations. Before reacting, ask yourself questions like *Is this situation the worst thing that could happen?* or *Am I making an assumption?* You could also ask yourself why you're upset by the situation. And remember, you may not be able to control the situation, but you can control and manage your judgments and perceptions, which is vital to reducing toxic structures in your brain and thereby reducing mental distress in your life.

27| Chase curiosity, not passion

It can be very stressful to focus just on "passion," as if it's a single, fixed thing. By focusing on finding the "one thing," you may miss out on so many other opportunities. It's sometimes better to follow what makes you curious, which often leads to passion. So, don't get stressed out if you don't have one thing you're passionate about and instead enjoy many different things, and don't judge others who keep trying new things and searching. Everyone's on a different path. What are you curious about today?

28| Start each morning by reminding yourself of three things

1 Life is short and can end at any moment. How would you like to spend your last moments?

2. Today will be a good day no matter what happens, because you can control your reactions. You can turn negative moments into learning opportunities.

3. One of the greatest human desires is to be relevant and connected. How can you help make someone feel relevant, connected, needed, and understood today?

29| Recognize the difference between reacting and responding

There's a major difference between reacting and responding. Reacting is often reflexive and impulsive, whereas responding is based on deliberate choice. Every day, we're given the opportunity either to react, where we can end up creating toxic thought patterns, negatively impacting our mental health, and damaging our relationships, or to learn to respond and control our reactions.

Responding requires gathering the facts first, taking time to think before speaking, and realizing that every thought or word creates a reality that will impact us and those around us. This gives us control, while just reacting gives someone or something else control over us. How can you start reacting less and responding more?

30| The most important conversations you have are with yourself

What do you say to yourself when no one's around? What world are you creating for yourself with your thoughts, words, and actions? Be honest with yourself and spend time each day gaining insight into how you think about and talk to yourself. You create your reality by the words you say and what you think, so awareness is vital.

31| What kind of advice do you give to others?

What advice do you give out the most? Pay attention to this, as it may be an indication of something you need to address in your own life.

32| Be vulnerable with those you love

If you struggle to be open and find it hard
to talk to people about your feelings, I
encourage you to be brave and vulnerable.
Take it one step at a time and embrace
the uncomfortableness and uncertainty.
Remember, it's far braver to acknowledge
emotions than to suppress them. Only
once you acknowledge your feelings can
you begin to heal.

33| Join a community

Research shows that the more we're involved in a social group, the less our risk of death is from all causes, while relationships of any kind can potentially improve our chances of survival by up to 50 percent. How can you become more involved in your community? Think of ways you can join a group and build up your social circle.

34| Freak out in the "love zone"

When something frustrating or bad happens and you need to vent, set a timer on your phone for five minutes. In those five minutes, scream, cry, yell, shout, and do whatever you need to do to get it all out. When those five minutes are done, force yourself to stop and say, "I can't control the events and circumstances of life, but I can control my reactions to them." This will help you move on and not fixate on the issue.

35| Do you criticize others?

Do you find yourself quick to judge and criticize? Often, we criticize change in someone because it forces us to confront something in our own life. Watch how you react to someone else's life, because this may be a signal you need to address something in your life.

36| Argue well

It is incredibly important to remember that, in any argument, it's not you against the other person. Rather, it's you and the other person against the issue. Separate the human from the problem.

37| Don't assume you know what someone is thinking or feeling

Assumptions are the mother of all mess-ups. Often, we make assumptions about someone's words or actions, and instead of asking for more information and clarification, we just get stuck thinking about what we thought we heard or saw. This thinking is often toxic and can cause mental distress. Save yourself the trouble and pain by asking for clarity and always questioning thoughts you have. *Are they true? Do I have all the facts? Am I misjudging or misreading this person or situation?* Just because you think something doesn't mean it's true.

38| Watch what you think and say about yourself

Be careful what labels you associate with your identity. Take a few moments today to look at how you label yourself and how you see yourself. Are you taking on any unnecessary titles? For example, instead of saying "my anxiety," you can say, "I am struggling with anxiety at the moment." Don't let your issues define who you are at your core, which can keep you locked in and prevent healing.

39| Don't celebrate the workaholic

We need to stop glorifying the person who works all weekend and start praising the person who finds a good work-life balance. Our culture of celebrating the workaholic is one of the main reasons why we're seeing an increase in mental, emotional, and physical burnout. Do you glorify work over relationships? Do you think how long you work defines your self-worth? Consider your relationship with work and how you can improve it.

40| Start and end the day right

As you wake up, tell yourself today will be a great day and discuss with yourself or a loved one *why* it will be great. And before you go to sleep, think about and discuss why your day was great. Doing this on a regular basis will train your brain to focus more on the positive; our expectations change the structure of our brain in a good way. How will you start your day off today?

41| Don't regret making mistakes in front of your children

As parents, we often feel guilty for making mistakes in front of our children. But we shouldn't try to cover up our faults or let our shame and guilt control us. Rather, we should reconceptualize our mistakes as invaluable teaching opportunities that will help prepare our children to successfully navigate the hard parts of life. We need to be brave enough to admit we're wrong and strong enough to fix the mistake and move on. We need to teach our children to be vulnerable, open, and honest, and model for them how to turn a mistake into an opportunity for growth.

42| Just because you think something, that doesn't mean it's true

When you find you are overthinking, anxious, angry, or experiencing any kind of toxic emotion, spend a few minutes examining your thoughts and see if they are true and factual. Are you making assumptions? Are you overexaggerating? Then check your thinking by talking to someone else to get perspective and more information. From there, decide to replace the untrue thought with the truth, which may not always be "nice." You may be the one responsible or at fault in a situation. However, it's better to face reality now than further build up toxic structures in your brain, which will become realities in your life and affect your mental health.

43| Learn how to manage stress

It's so vital to learn how to correctly react to and manage stress, as this will help develop mental toughness and build up your stress resilience, which, in turn, will help you deal with stressful situations in the future. Make a game plan so that you'll know what to do when you're stressed about something. The more you practice reacting to stressful situations in a good way, the more you are strengthening healthy memories in your brain and building up your mental immunity.

44| Define your own success

When you don't define your own success, the world will define it for you. When was the last time you really thought long and hard about what success meant for you in your own life? Take a few moments today to write down what success in your personal, professional, spiritual, physical, mental, and emotional life looks like, and really reflect on what you wrote. Be sure to revisit what you wrote periodically to check if you're on track. Remember to be flexible in the exact details and how you'll get there.

45| Don't just wait for life to give you what you want

Don't live with the mindset of just expecting things from life. Rather, have a mindset that asks, *What is life expecting from me?* The first attitude removes responsibility from the individual and is more likely to cause disillusionment, anxiety from lack of control, and other mental health issues. The second attitude gives control back to the individual, as well as more responsibility. In my practice and research, I've seen that those who feel like they have more control over their lives and decisions struggle less with mental ill-health. So, make it a habit to ask yourself, *What is life expecting of me? Can I do better? How can I be more responsible for my choices, actions, and thoughts?*

46| Make "gathering time" an important part of your life

Be intentional about creating moments in your day or week when you can just sit, reflect, and be by yourself. I call these moments "gathering time," and they are vital for your mental health. Use this time to be self-reflective, journal, learn something new, meditate, pray, or just simply daydream. I highly recommend scheduling these moments into your calendar so you don't forget to do them or give up that time. I've found that these moments often show me where my thinking is toxic and what bad habits I need to work on.

47| Use your free time to build your brain

Make it a habit to use the free moments in your day to build your brain and increase your knowledge. Free moments can be when you're getting ready, driving, walking, waiting for an appointment, and so on. Instead of getting on social media, read a book or listen to a podcast, TED interview, or audiobook. Be intentional every day about how you use free moments, because these few moments add up to hours and hours a year.

48| Don't be afraid to argue

One hour of arguing correctly can save years of relationship problems. We need to stop fearing arguments and sweeping things "under the rug" and start learning how to argue correctly. Only when we get everything out can we begin to find the core issues and also find healing—mentally, physically, and emotionally—in relationships.

49| What kind of language do you use?

Does the language you use put people on the defensive? It's so important to watch how you phrase things and what words you choose. Avoid statements such as "You're *always* ____" and "You *never* ____." Also avoid assigning blame. Try looking inward and asking yourself if you're partly responsible for the situation. Is there an underlying issue you're not addressing? Arguing can be so good for relationships if done correctly. One key tip is to learn to speak in ways that don't trigger or aggravate others.

50| Don't avoid hard tasks

The longer you push aside an unpleasant task, the more time you have to think about it, making it something even more unpleasant and stressful. Make it a habit to get it done first thing so it doesn't cause you mental distress. This will reduce the anxiety or stress associated with this task and help improve your mental health. What can you get done today that you have been putting off for a while?

51| Take measures against cognitive decline

Do you worry about cognitive decline? Or maybe you know someone who has it and want to know how to help? One of the best ways to prevent the onset or worsening of cognitive decline is to improve both short- and long-term memory. This builds up the cognitive reserves in the brain, which are more and more important as you age. To strengthen your short-term memory, practice memorizing shopping lists, phone numbers, passwords, poems, songs, and so on. To strengthen your long-term memory, spend at least an hour a day building your brain through deep, intellectual thinking and learning: read educational books, listen to a podcast on something new and interesting, and reteach what you have learned to a friend or family member.

52| Reach out and help others when you are feeling down

Part of a good mental self-care regimen is reaching out and helping others, even if we're struggling with our own issues. Too often we get stuck trying to deal with our own problems, which can make us self-absorbed and make our issues worse: our problems get larger because they are all we see. Helping others, on the other hand, not only boosts our own healing but is a great way to gain perspective and gratitude and build up our mental toughness. Sometimes the best remedy is getting out of our head and helping others.

53| Be proactive in building human connections

Don't expect people to instantly connect with you. Don't put the responsibility on others. Take the time to analyze the quality of your connections and how you can improve your relationships. One great way to proactively build meaningful connections with someone is to take interest in what they like (even if it doesn't particularly appeal to you). Ask questions, listen, do research, put aside judgment, and embrace curiosity. Human connection is one of the best antidepressants.

54| Don't panic if you can't fall asleep

Don't allow yourself to lie in bed panicking about not sleeping. Instead, get excited and embrace the fact you're awake. Tell yourself, *This is going to be a nice, quiet time when I'm not bugged by texts, emails, or people needing something. I'm going to get that research done, finally read that book, watch that program on the Discovery Channel, tidy that closet, or work uninterrupted on that project!* This excitement lowers cortisol levels, balances the HPA axis (the "stress axis"), and makes stress work for you and not against you, activating your resilience and changing your genes in a good way. Develop a positive expectation that this is a special time just for you, and you will use it wisely. This mindset will help you get your panic under control and improve your health. A mindset of negative expectation, however, is just going to damage your brain and make you feel worse—it's not worth it!

55| Anticipating the worst moments creates the worst moments

When we anticipate or expect the worst to happen, we build that thinking into our brain, which can affect our actions, attitudes, and words. Remember, your expectations create realities. Remind yourself that bad days or weeks won't last forever, and plan to celebrate when they're over. Let the anticipation of a reward help you enjoy the process of facing the day's or week's challenges.

56| Focus on the "now"

When it comes to tough times, it is so important to focus on the "now" moment (the present). Don't fear or dread the future, and don't ruminate on the past, especially past failures and mistakes. When we focus too much on future fears and worries, we lose sight of what is happening now and how to make the "now" work for us and not against us. Also, focusing on the past keeps us stuck there, unable to deal with the now or even enjoy the present moment. By fearing the future or regretting the past, we reinforce those neural networks in our brain and can create mental chaos. In the midst of a bad day or week, focus on the present: What can you do to make the situation work for you right now, what can you learn, and what is your mindset?

57| Don't downgrade the seriousness of someone else's struggles

How many times have you heard someone say, "Oh, it's not that bad," or "So-and-so is stressed, but they don't know what real stress is," or "You think you're stressed? I'm so overwhelmed!"? These kinds of statements are very dangerous; they demonstrate a sense of self-involvement and a lack of compassion and understanding for others. You will never know the degree of pain or stress someone else is in because you're not the one feeling it. So, practice empathy and always do your best to hear what someone's trying to tell you in a nonjudgmental way.

58| When dealing with difficult people, sometimes it's best to build trust first

When dealing with someone who is difficult and doesn't want help or seems to not want to change, sometimes the best approach is to first build trust and a stronger relationship by engaging with them on topics they're interested in and listening to them without judgment. Don't just try to solve their issues! This doesn't mean you ignore the problem; rather, you go into a conversation or interaction wanting to engage with that person on topics that interest them, building up trust, which is the foundation for true change. Doing this will help facilitate deep and meaningful conversations in the future and can make the person more receptive to what you have to say (you don't want your words to feel like a sudden intervention).

59| Appreciate the journey of life

As you go about your day, don't just focus on how much you can get done. Rather, focus on how much you can *learn*. Life has so much to offer—embrace it!

60| Don't judge a book by its cover

It's always important to realize there's a deeper message below someone's outward actions and words. Focus on that rather than on "So-and-so did this," especially in difficult situations. Keep in mind the *bigger picture*: Why do you care about this person? Think about the love you have for your friend or family member.

61 | Get your mind in order before you go to sleep

The secret to better sleep isn't some pill. Rather, it's consistent mental self-care and mind management. If your mind's in chaos, no pill or sleeping trick will work. It's important to remember that there is no quick fix for detoxing your mind and brain; it's a *lifestyle*. This is basic mental self-care, as necessary as bathing and cleaning your teeth. It keeps your brain healthy and heals the damage from toxic thinking, which may be contributing to keeping you awake at night.

62| Protect your own mental health when dealing with difficult people

Throughout the whole process of dealing with a difficult person, you need to remember to protect your own mental health, because these kinds of situations can be tough and draining. Make sure you have a designated person you can talk to who can help you process difficult situations and emotions. And, where applicable, use technology to your advantage: if a difficult person calls but you need a rest, let it go to voicemail and text them that you will call back later. Sometimes it's better to text rather than call; it can help you think clearly before responding in a reactive and emotional way. Indeed, always take the time to think before you respond—never react impulsively! And when you do feel attacked, imagine a shield of armor around your mind protecting you from the "arrows" of their nasty words. This can help you divorce your own emotions from the issue and give your mind a break by reminding yourself it's just their pain speaking, not a direct attack on you. It's important to set *definitive boundaries*!

63| Make "mental autopsies" a regular part of your day

When you are dealing with a difficult situation or person or just an overall bad day, conduct a "mental autopsy." Look back at your past experiences, analyze them, and examine why something went the way it did and how you can improve, whether this is some kind of trauma, a fight, an issue at work, or something similar. Mental autopsies are conducted after a mistake or experience in order to see what went wrong (or right), just as a regular autopsy looks at a dead body to see what went wrong. The key to a good mental autopsy is *understanding*. When you start to understand your experiences, you can reconceptualize them (or redesign them) and learn from them, instead of overthinking and making the same mistakes repeatedly. Ask, answer, and discuss with yourself why something happened, how it happened, what the triggers were, and so on. This will help you gain insight into the issue and see how it can be avoided in the future or how you can improve the way you react the next time something similar happens.

64 | Make mental plans of what you want to change or achieve

When it comes to creating sustainable habits in your life, planning and writing down your goals in a way that enables you to see the big picture and remind yourself of it on a daily basis is incredibly important. Journaling and using a calendar, habit tracker, or something similar can be helpful. Writing things down helps organize your thinking, which, in turn, helps you make better decisions because you can stand outside yourself and observe your life from a more "neutral" and less emotional vantage point. Have a clear vision of why and what you want to change.

65| If someone you know is struggling, listen to their story

If you know someone who is suffering from depression or anxiety, don't just reach out to them to try "fix" them. Simply connect with them and listen and tune in to their needs and their unique story. People want to be heard, not corrected or "fixed."

66| Teach your children that feeling sad or anxious isn't wrong

Parents and guardians: teach your children that anxiety and depression are normal parts of life and will come and go. These feelings don't mean that your children are "broken" or that something is wrong with them. Overprotecting your children won't prepare them for the toughness of life. Teach them how to wrestle with the hard parts of life and how to make it through tough times. Show them how to be resilient by demonstrating your love for

them through your words and actions, and
be open with them about your own struggles.
Create an environment where your children
can talk to you without judgment.

67| Recognize that material objects aren't everything

Our enjoyment from material things will always decline over time. Keep this in mind the next time you are tempted to think an object you desire will bring lasting happiness.

68| Think about happiness differently

Happiness isn't a fixed state or something that's definable or quantifiable. Happiness isn't perpetual feelings of joy or euphoria. It's not a consumer product. It's not found or discovered. Happiness is generated by us through the way we frame and manage the events of life and our expectations of these events. There's no secret to happiness. Remember, you don't find happiness, *you create it*.

69| Learn to handle rejection

When faced with rejection, don't immediately think there's something wrong with you. Rather, objectify the situation, assuming the role of an inspector or detective, and examine what happened from an impartial position. This will help take the sting out of the situation and allow you to find clarity and turn the situation into a learning experience.

70| Watch what you think

Your mind controls your brain, and your brain controls your body. If you want a healthy body, you need a healthy mind. Physical change starts with a mental change. You are—and you become—what you *think*.

71| Practice doing nothing

Many of us feel guilty when we need to take a break or holiday because we live in a society that constantly tells us we are only valuable if we work all the time. We overvalue people who work overtime, glorifying their hectic schedules, and undervalue the power and beauty of rest and relaxation. We need to recognize that although the mind is infinite, the brain is finite, and it needs rest to function well. We can give our best only when we are rested, which is why it is so important to learn how to be okay with doing nothing from time to time, even if it is just for a few minutes. How can you practice doing "nothing" today?

72| Be a peacemaker, not a people-pleaser

Are you a people-pleaser or peacemaker?
A *peacemaker* seeks to restore balance
and find a resolution—and is other-
focused. A *people-pleaser*, on the other
hand, is self-focused, often wishing to
avoid conflict and uncertainty to the point
of sacrificing their mental health and
morals.

73| Adopt a curiosity mindset

Try this the next time you're dealing with someone who's being rude or angry: calmly ask for more details and an explanation for why they're angry or why they're frustrated with you, rather than just reacting. This mindset will change your body language and tone of voice, which may help soothe the other person, forcing them to pause and think before attacking you.

74| Change the way you value yourself

Don't base your self-worth on the number of tasks you can complete in a day. Base your self-worth on how you have grown and what you have learned in a day.

75| Listen to your body and stop overthinking

How do you know whether you're overthinking or thinking deeply? Your body and mind will tell you. When you're overthinking, you will step into toxic stress and your body will respond—maybe you'll feel sick or get a headache. It's also important to analyze your thinking and emotions so you can find out what's making you overthink and deal with the cause. Ask yourself why you feel stressed about something, what is actually happening, how you can change the situation, and how your mindset is affecting your ability to deal with it. Write down your thoughts; this can bring clarity to the situation at hand. Turn overthinking into *deep thinking*.

76| Ask for clarification if you're overthinking a situation

If you find yourself overthinking a situation or problem, take the time to ask the other person involved for more clarification before making assumptions that will only lead to more overthinking. Ask them what they mean, why they said what they said, or why they did what they did. Be sure to calm down before angrily or reactively snapping back. Be patient. Asking for more information will definitely help avoid misunderstandings that come as a result of miscommunication.

77| Choose not to be oversensitive

It's very important not to overthink
situations or assume that people have
said or acted in a certain way because
they were trying to antagonize you. Do
not victimize yourself. Choose to stop and
think about the situation in a rational way,
and don't let your emotions get the best
of you. Examine how you see yourself,
write it down, and think of ways you can
give people the benefit of the doubt
rather than just assuming you know their
thoughts.

78| Make it a priority to spend at least an hour a day reading

Not only does reading build the brain in a healthy way but it also helps develop our mirror neurons and people skills. It opens up the parts of the brain responsible for our compassion, understanding, and empathy, making us better leaders, teachers, parents, and siblings.

79| Take measures to prevent overeating

Overeating can have a negative impact on your physical *and* mental health. To prevent overeating, try to wait twenty minutes before getting a second helping of food. Maybe have a cup of coffee or tea or go for a walk. This will allow your brain to "catch up" to your stomach and recognize how full you are. If you eat too quickly and with too many distractions (TV, phone, eating on the go), your brain can miss the signal from your stomach that you are full.

80 | Change the way you react to negative feedback

No one likes receiving negative feedback— we feel attacked or embarrassed. Instead of lashing out, however, take a few seconds to calm down. Think about what the person said and measure your response. Say something like, "I appreciate you taking the time and effort to tell me that. Thank you." This will make you more open to feedback in the future, which can help you improve, grow, and learn.

81| Keep an "unease" journal

One way of identifying what is causing you anxiety and mental distress is to keep a record of moments when you feel uneasy. Write down the details of the situation, what your triggers could be, how you felt, and who you were with. Much like a food journal can be helpful when it comes to identifying allergies and intolerances, an "unease" journal can help you identify issues you need to deal with.

82| Become aware of the problems in your life

Awareness of a problem is great. Although it may not feel great to be aware of something bad in your life, it is an incredibly important part of the healing process. Only once you're aware of an issue can you begin to change it. How often have you brushed aside a feeling of sadness or loneliness without taking a look at why you feel that way? Issues cannot be suppressed for long. Celebrate being aware, then move on and take action to remedy the situation. What problems can you become aware of and start changing in your life?

83| Don't be afraid to admit you are jealous

Jealousy is something no one likes to admit, yet it is a dangerous emotion and needs to be dealt with immediately. Jealousy causes damage in the brain and can contribute to mental ill-health. So, what's the first step to dealing with jealousy? Admit it. Embrace the ugliness. Only then can you begin to change. Spend some time today and ask yourself if you have any jealousy in your life.

84| Don't be discouraged if the journey is taking longer than expected

It takes twenty-one days to build a new long-term memory and sixty-three days to build a new habit. What's the moral of the story? Change takes time, so don't get discouraged if you don't see results immediately. Also, be wary of anyone who promises a quick fix to a problem—any results will only be temporary. True and lasting change takes time.

85| Make gratitude a priority today and every day

Always be grateful. There are people who would love to have your bad day. Gratitude makes us feel that life is worth living, which brings mental health benefits in a positive feedback loop leading to more resilience— the ability to bounce back more quickly during hard times. Gratitude is therefore essential to overcoming difficult circumstances and achieving success in all areas of your life.

86| Smile and laugh often

Remember to smile often and fill your life
with moments of humor. Research shows
that smiling and laughter can boost the
immune system, ease pain, relax the body,
and even reduce the effects of negative
stress.

87| Daydream often

You've probably had someone in your life tell you to stop daydreaming. Well, I'm here to tell you daydreaming is actually very good for you! Letting your mind wander gives your brain a physical rest and allows the free flow of information, which helps combat negative thinking patterns while boosting creativity and imagination. So, take a few seconds each day to just let your thoughts drift!

88| Change the way you see a stressful situation

Did you know stress can be good for you?
When you view a stressful situation as an
unconquerable mountain, you shift into
toxic stress. However, if you change your
attitude about a stressful situation, you can
also change the outcome. A good reaction
to stress keeps you alert and can increase
cognitive function and flexibility. Remember,
the way you view a situation will determine
how you deal with that situation, so
choose to be positive and see challenges as
opportunities to grow and learn.

89| Replace negative, toxic thoughts with an "attitude of gratitude"

Every time you find yourself feeling down, think about all the good things in your life. This will change the brain and body for the better: gratitude can increase your longevity, your ability to use your imagination, and your ability to problem-solve. So, when you're at a low point in life, write down what you're grateful for on a sticky note and place it somewhere near you. Perhaps text or call a friend and tell them how thankful you are to have them in your life. Remember, the more good you see in your life in the now moments, the happier and more successful you're likely to be at school, work, and life in the future.

90| Don't spend too much time defining the problem

When it comes to any situation we face, we often spend too much time focusing on the problem and too little time focusing on the solution. Essentially, we can be quite good at recognizing what we need to change but not the how or when. In fact, if we spend too much time ruminating on the problem, we can get caught up in the emotions associated with the toxic thinking pattern, which can lead to emotional burnout, mental fatigue, and increased anxiety. When dealing with a situation, or just life in general, it's best to spend a limited amount of time defining what the issue is and focus more time on a plan of action. So, the next time you find yourself faced with a challenge, think of different ways a situation can work to your benefit. I personally try to stick with a "one-third plan" when it comes to dealing with a negative thinking pattern or a stressful situation: I use one-third of my time to define and talk about the issue, one-third to plan the solution, and one-third to transform the solution into some kind of positive action.

91| Don't make decisions when you're tired

The brain has limited energy and needs recharging. We do this through lifestyle choices like good nutrition and exercise, but, even more so, with good mind-management techniques. Our mind is infinite and tireless; our brain is finite and gets tired. When it's tired, chemicals don't flow like they should, and the internal networks of the brain can get stuck or overfire. This is akin to driving through a storm with broken windshield wipers—a recipe for disaster. It is important to take regular mental health breaks throughout the day, in the form of "thinker moments," to daydream for a few moments; I recommend a minute or so every hour. These moments give your brain a rest and allow it to reboot and heal, increasing your clarity of thought and organizing the networks of your brain, which will help you make wise decisions instead of "shooting from the hip."

92| Have a "possibilities mindset"

We need to be realistic, of course, but we also need to have what I call a "possibilities mindset." If we just assume we've failed because things haven't gone our way, we can block ourselves from moving forward, which can upset our mental well-being because our brain gets stuck in a negative, stressful reaction. However, when we learn to think that there's more than just plan A or plan B, we tap into the optimism bias of the brain, which helps us get up when we fail, and we don't get stressed out when things don't go as planned. Being prepared to change our thoughts in this way, especially when our circumstances change, helps develop mental flexibility, resilience, creativity, and imagination, which gives us hope because we just keep on trying until we achieve our goals! So, practice seeing multiple possibilities in any given situation, maybe even writing them down in your journal.

93| Have a strong support system in place

Each time you feel yourself teetering on the brink of toxic stress, speak with your friends or family (even if it is just a phone call or text conversation) to help get perspective and deal with your anxiety in a positive way. Finding life difficult at times isn't something to be ashamed of, while suppressing your emotions will throw your brain and body into toxic stress, which can severely impact your mental and physical health. This is why it's so important to develop a habit of reaching out when times get tough. It helps strengthen your brain's immunity to stress by activating positive genetic switches in the brain. *Remember, the key to dealing with stress is not pretending you're always okay; rather, resilience to stress comes from being proactive in seeking help and helping others.*

94| Don't get stuck in a victim mentality

It's very important to avoid a victim mentality, which can keep us stuck in toxic stress reactions and decrease our resilience to stressful situations. When we take responsibility for our choices and our life, we can feel more in control and recognize that although we can't control other people's thoughts or reactions, we can control our own thoughts and actions. So, watch what you say and think about what happens in your life. Do you always feel like a victim? Do you take responsibility for your choices?

95| Work on your self-confidence

Spend time discovering what you're good at. What do you love? What makes you want to get out of bed in the morning and take on the world? Read more books on all kinds of topics to discover what interests you and think about times you were happiest or at peace and re-create those times. This will help you be at peace with who you are and who you want to be, regardless of what other people think about you. In fact, thinking about your relationships with friends or other loved ones with whom you're happy and can be yourself can help you learn to see yourself in a positive light. Write this down! We all have something great to give to the world. Learn to respect and harness this greatness, which will help intrinsically motivate you to be the best version of yourself you can be, and you will not be driven by extrinsic factors such as what someone else thinks about you.

96| Focus on healthy habits, not quick-fix solutions

When it comes to your health, you need to focus on long-term goals, not quick fixes or sudden solutions. When we try to cheat our own biology with extreme diets or programs, we may get to our goals in a short amount of time—but we could also be doing untold damage to our brain and body. It's much more beneficial to spend time building healthy habits. Focusing on this process rather than some unrealistic goal builds a strong mental foundation for true change by strengthening your character through self-examination and discipline. As you turn your attention toward cultivating a mindset and attitude that enjoys the process of getting healthy, you can actually build and develop good, long-term mental habits. So, rather than going from one diet to the next, it's far better to work at developing a healthy lifestyle that will allow you to succeed in the long term, one which incorporates healthy thinking, eating, sleeping, and exercise habits. When you adopt this big-picture approach to your physical health, you can truly focus on improving every area of your life and sustaining patterns of behavior that help you live your best life.

97| Step up to the challenge

Challenges can bring out the best in us. Getting to the other side of a challenge brings a sense of happiness in the achievement, toughening the mind and setting the stage for the next challenge with the addition of the new skills we have gained. Mental training via deep thinking and understanding to build memory and learning increases the numbers of neurons that develop in the brain, particularly when the training goals are challenging. This growth of neurons with their dendrites (where memory is actually stored) means long-term, useful, and meaningful memories are formed, thereby toughening the mind and forming the basis for success. Choose to do something every day that challenges your mind, whether it's reading a book, learning a language, or studying something that interests you. Plan ahead and choose something that will help you expand your knowledge base and develop self-discipline and mental resilience.

98| Stop comparing yourself to others

Comparison is a killer, plain and simple. It will impact how you think about your own abilities and affect your capacity to use your mind to succeed in school, the workplace, and life. It's important to remind yourself that the law of the brain is diversity: there's no "normal" human, and if you try be an Einstein or a Céline Dion, you will fail. You make a lousy someone else but a perfect you, because you think in a completely unique and wonderful way. It's up to you, therefore, to design your own blueprint for success. You can do

something no one else in the world can do—
now that is something to celebrate! Develop
an *expectancy mindset* when you think about
yourself: expect great things. Perhaps write
what you love to do and want to do in a
journal and read it when you feel low.

99| Set work boundaries

Sometimes, we have to work hard on a deadline or something urgent needs to get done while we are on holiday. If this is the case, it is important to set work boundaries by budgeting an amount of time during the day to work, and then stopping and resting when it is done (using the timer or alarm on your phone can be helpful). Don't just say, "Let me finish this quick," because you may end up working for hours on things that really don't need to get done; schedule work like you would schedule a lunch date, and then enjoy your time off!

100| Focus on your journey

Compare yourself to how you were yesterday, not to how someone else is today. Everyone's journey is unique. Don't focus on what someone else is doing and envy that, because you'll never be that person. Concentrate on improving each day, even if it's small improvements. Maybe try working out a bit more each day or spend a bit more time reading and learning a new skill each day. Focus on your journey.

101| Write a gratitude letter to someone in your life

When was the last time you wrote a letter just thanking someone for being in your life? This is one of the easiest things you can do to boost your mental health. Studies have shown that this simple act will not only enhance your own happiness and well-being but also strengthen meaningful relationships in your life, since writing a letter shows you're willing to invest time in your relationship with that person.

conclusion

Everyone seems to be talking about mindfulness and taking the time to invest in yourself. Well, you have gone *beyond* mindfulness in using this book. You have started learning how to make your mind work *for you*—how to use your mind to shape your life. You're investing in your mental self-care and creating a lifestyle that promotes brain and body health.

You've started learning how to go beyond being aware of your thoughts, calming down, and acknowledging your feelings, thoughts, and bodily sensations in the present moment.

You've learned how to manage your response in the moment and make sustainable, long-lasting changes. You are the "captain of your soul."

The thing you need to always remember is that you have significant resources at your fingertips: *your mind is incredibly powerful*. You can use your thoughts to improve your overall intellect, cognitive performance, and mental and physical well-being. Harnessing these natural resources will give you power over your present, depth and context to your past, and anticipation for the future.

about the author

DR. CAROLINE LEAF is a communication pathologist and cognitive neuroscientist whose passion is to help people see the power of the mind to change the brain and find their purpose in life. She is the author of *Switch On Your Brain, Think and Eat Yourself Smart, The Perfect You,* and *Think, Learn, Succeed,* among many other books and journal articles, and her videos, podcasts, and TV episodes have reached millions globally. She currently teaches at various academic, medical, and neuroscience conferences, as well as in churches around the world. Dr. Leaf and her husband, Mac, live with their four children in Dallas and Los Angeles.

Live a **Happier, Healthier** Life

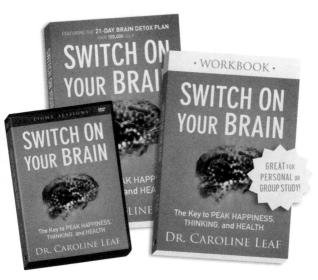

The bestselling book that has taught thousands
how to achieve and maintain optimal levels of
intelligence, mental health, peace, and happiness!

Tired of FAD DIETS, EMOTIONAL EATING, or POOR HEALTH?

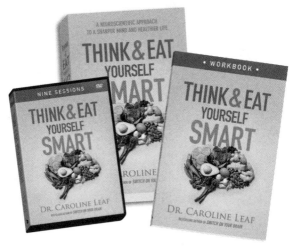

In this revolutionary book, Dr. Caroline Leaf packs an incredible amount of information that will change your eating and thinking habits for the better. Rather than getting caught up in fads, Leaf reveals that every individual has unique nutritional needs and there's no one perfect solution. Rather, she shows how to change the way you think about food and put yourself on the path toward health.

UNLOCK YOUR
HIDDEN POTENTIAL

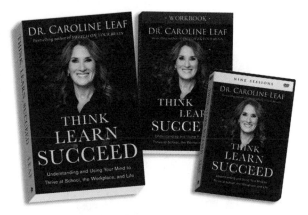

Backed by up-to-date scientific research and biblical insight, Dr. Caroline Leaf empowers readers to take control of their thoughts in order to take control of their lives. In this practical book, readers will learn to use

- The 5-Step Switch On Your Brain Learning Program, to build memory and learn effectively.
- The Gift Profile, to discover the unique way they process information.
- The Mindfulness Guide, to optimize their thought life and find their inner resilience.

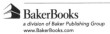

A HAPPIER, HEALTHIER, MORE ENJOYABLE LIFE— STARTING TODAY!

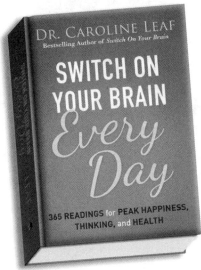

In her bestselling book *Switch On Your Brain*, Dr. Caroline Leaf offered a prescription for better health and wholeness through correct thinking patterns. Now she shows you how to instill the practices for living a healthy, happy life into your daily routine. These readings offer encouragement and strategies to reap the benefits of a detoxed thought life—every day!

Connect with
CAROLINE

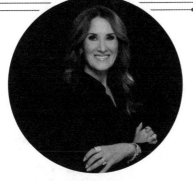

VISIT
DrLeaf.com

to learn more about Dr. Leaf and her
research, read her blog, listen to her podcast,
and follow her speaking schedule!

Also follow her on social media.

 drleaf

DrCarolineLeaf

drcarolineleaf

Dr. Caroline Leaf

DETOX YOUR BRAIN IN
21 DAYS!

—

DR. CAROLINE LEAF

sw**i**tch

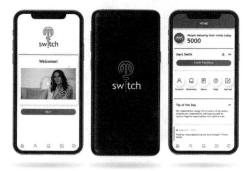

Eliminate stress, anxiety, depression, and toxic thinking with the **first ever brain detox app!**

SWITCH uses Dr. Leaf's scientifically researched and revolutionary SWITCH On Your Brain 5-Step Process® to help you take back control over your thoughts and your life.

VISIT THESWITCH.APP FOR MORE INFORMATION
OR DOWNLOAD ON THE APP STORE OR GOOGLE PLAY

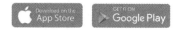

A TOP MENTAL HEALTH PODCAST
AROUND THE WORLD

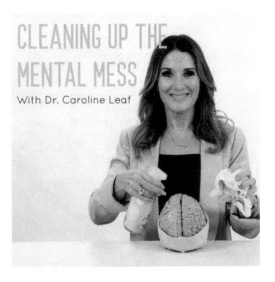

Tune in for practical tips and tools to help you take back control over your mental, emotional, and physical health.

Listen on Spotify, iTunes, PodBean, Anchor, YouTube, or DrLeaf.com.

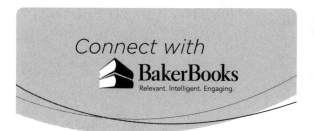
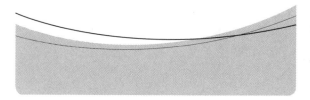
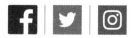